New Parents

BABY HACKS

Tips and Tricks Manual for Infants Care.

By CYNTHIA LEONARD

TABLE OF CONTENTS

About This Book

Congratulations on starting one of the most fulfilling adventures of your life: becoming a parent!

You're probably bursting with pleasure and love as you bring your little one into the world, but you're also probably a little nervous. You are not alone, so don't worry. Every parent goes through a range of emotions while navigating the wonderful turmoil that is parenting a kid.

We've put together a gold mine of priceless hints, techniques and hacks in this book to help you settle into this new phase of your life more easily. Taking care of a newborn may provide both exciting and intimidating difficulties, regardless of whether you're a first-time parent or are expanding your family.

We can help with everything from resolving restless nights to handling feeding issues, from understanding the art of calming a fussy infant to interpreting their screams. Using the combined knowledge of paediatricians, child development specialists and seasoned parents, we've put together a thorough handbook that tackles frequent issues and offers workable answers.

However, the focus of this work is flourishing rather than only surviving. We want to provide you the tools you need to confidently and joyfully embrace every one of the many amazing moments that come with becoming a parent. Learning to navigate the ups and downs of motherhood can be enjoyable and gratifying if you have a little imagination, ingenuity, and humour.

For that reason, **"New Parents - Baby Hacks"** is here to help you every step of the way, whether you're looking for techniques for changing diapers, ideas for creating a bedtime routine or just a comforting voice in the middle of the turmoil.

Together, let's set out on this journey to discover the keys to becoming the greatest parent you can be.

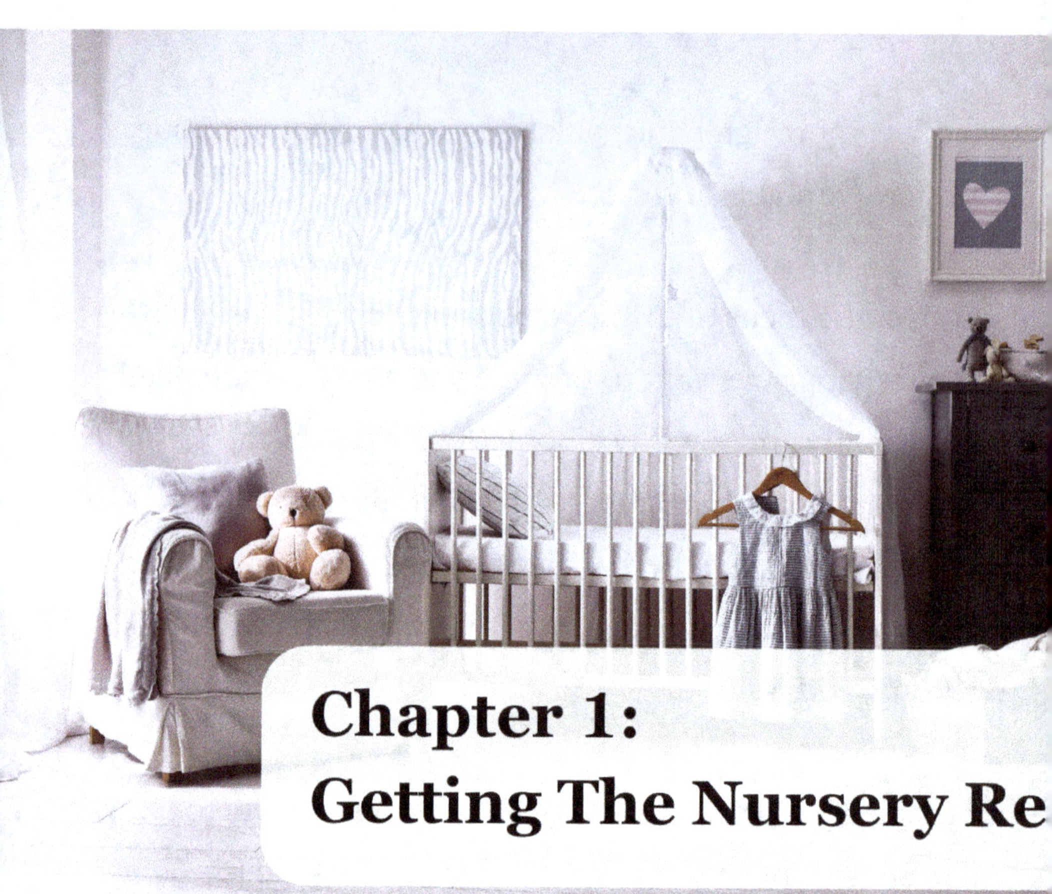

Getting The Nursery Ready:

Since your baby's cot will serve as the focal point of their sleeping space, selecting the ideal cot for your nursery is a crucial choice. When choosing a cot, take into account the following important factors:

Verify that the cot complies with the most recent safety regulations. Cribs need, for instance, adhere to Consumer Product Safety Commission **(CPSC)** regulations in the United States. To make sure the cot satisfies safety regulations, look for certification markings like those from the American Society for Testing and Materials (ASTM) or the Juvenile Products Manufacturers Association (JPMA).

Robust Construction: In order to provide your infant a safe resting environment, the cot has to be well-built with solid materials. Look for any sharp edges or loose items that can injure your youngster.

Mattress Fit: There should be only **two fingers'** worth of space between the mattress and the crib edges so that the mattress fits snugly within the crib. This reduces the possibility of being trapped or suffocating.

Adjustable Mattress Height: Keep an eye out for cribs that provide mattress height adjustments. With the help of this feature, you can lessen the chance of your baby climbing or falling out of the cot as they become bigger and more active.

Convertible Options: Take into account cribs with features that can be converted into a toddler bed, daybed or even a full-sized bed. This may add value over time and increase the crib's lifetime as your kid gets older.

Style and Design: Select a cot based on your particular style choices and the décor of your nursery. There are many different kinds of cribs, including convertible, sleigh, contemporary and classic designs. Take into account elements like colour, polish and visual appeal.

Budget: Establish a spending limit and look for cribs that fit into that range. Don't forget to account for extra expenses for things like a mattress, bedding and other necessary accessories.

Reviews and Advice: Go over what other parents have to say about the cribs you're considering and ask relatives and friends who have recently bought cribs for advice. Their knowledge and perspectives may assist you in reaching a well-informed choice.

Space Considerations: Measure your nursery's size to make sure the cot will fit snugly without taking up too much room. Think about the other pieces of furniture and décor you want to add to the space.

Ease of Assembly and Maintenance: Find out how simple it is to construct and maintain the cot by reading reviews or product specs. Look for characteristics like simple assembly instructions and smooth surfaces that are easy to clean.

By taking these things into account, you can choose a cot that gives your infant a secure, cosy and fashionable place to sleep while also giving you, as a parent, peace of mind.

Organise Baby's Clothes

To organise your baby's wardrobe, divide clothing by size, sort by season and use storage options like drawers or boxes.

* Hang bulkier items like coats, dresses and jackets.
* Fold smaller items like onesies, pyjamas and slacks into drawers or shelves.
* Sort related items together to make finding necessary pieces easier.
* Label boxes or drawers with specific names for easy access.

Rotate your wardrobe as needed as your child grows, discarding unfit items and replacing them with larger and more suitable clothing.

Store special occasion attire separately and name them with the occasion and size. If your child outgrows certain items, donate them to a good cause or give them to relatives or friends with smaller children.

This practical and orderly system will help you keep their wardrobe clutter-free and make dressing your baby easier.

Setting Up a Diaper Changing Station

To ensure your baby's comfort and safety during diaper changes, you must set up a changing station in your nursery. *Below is a step-by-step guidance to assist you in creating a practical and useful space for changing diapers:*

Choose a Location: Choose a place in the nursery that is easy to get to and provides plenty room to move about. For easier cleaning, it's ideal to choose a location near a water supply.

Purchase a solid Changing Table or Pad: This may be as simple as placing a changing pad on top of a dresser or other solid surface. In order to keep your infant safe when changing diapers, make sure the table or pad has safety straps.

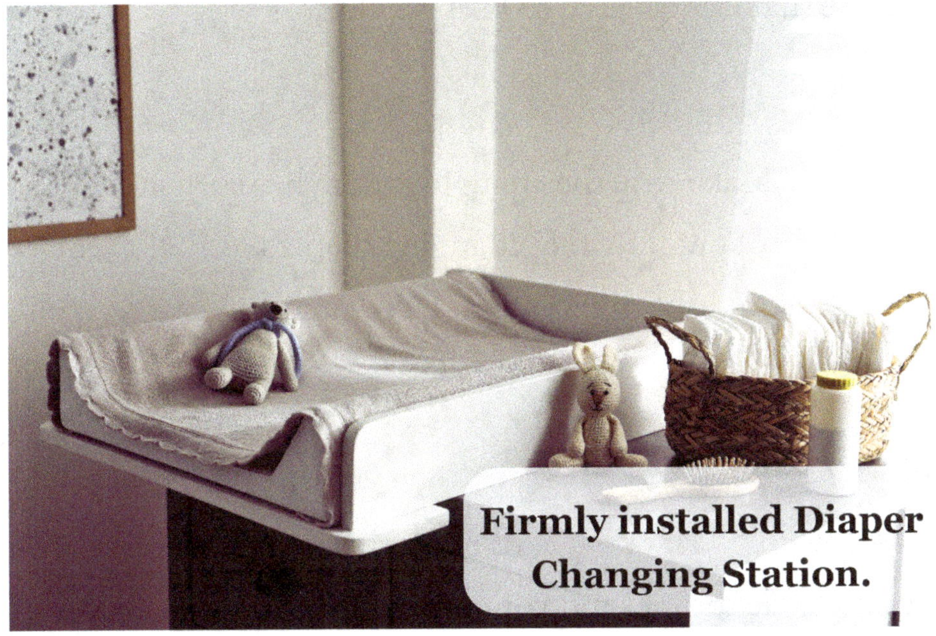

Arrange Materials: Compile all required materials and arrange them in an accessible manner. This contains changing pad covers, hand sanitizer, diaper rash treatment, wipes, diapers and one outfit change for your infant.

Storage Ideas: To keep the materials properly arranged and conveniently accessible, use organisers, boxes or baskets. For added convenience, think about adding shelves or storage spaces to the changing table.

Trash Bin: To make it simple to get rid of old wipes and diapers, put a little trash can next to the changing area. Ensure that it is covered to keep smells in.

Lighting: Make sure the changing room has enough light, particularly at night while changing diapers. A nightlight or a gentle, adjustable light may aid in establishing a peaceful environment.

Comfortable Mat or Rug: To make the changing area more comfortable for you and your infant, place a soft, machine-washable mat or rug below it.

Safety precautions: To avoid mishaps, install safety locks on cupboards and drawers that are within your baby's reach. Keep any potentially dangerous things out of your baby's reach, including sharp objects and drugs.

Personal Touches: To make the changing station seem cosier, add unique elements like wall decals, framed pictures or a mobile suspended above the changing table.

Keep it Clean: To keep your baby's surroundings tidy and sanitary, clean the changing area on a regular basis. Use a mild cleaning solution to clean the changing table, pad and around surfaces.

Create a Comfortable Feeding Area and Install Blackout Curtains for Better Sleep.

COMFORTABLE FEEDING AREA:
To create a comfortable feeding area, choose a quiet corner in the nursery and consider proximity to a power outlet.

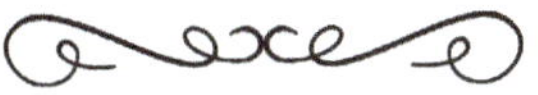

Invest in a rocking chair, glider or armchair with supportive cushions and armrests for long feeding sessions.

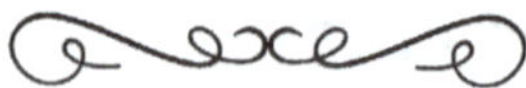

Use a footrest or ottoman for foot support and maintain a comfortable position.

Place a small side table next to the chair to hold essentials like burp cloths, water bottles, snacks and a lamp for nighttime lighting.

Add storage baskets or shelves for extra blankets and supplies. Decorate the area with soothing colours, textures and personal touches to create a calming atmosphere.

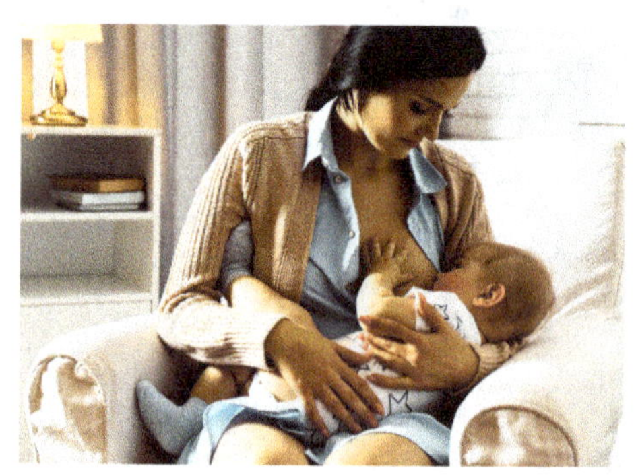

BLACKOUT CURTAINS FOR BETTER SLEEP:
To improve sleep in a nursery, measure the window dimensions and choose high-quality blackout curtains made from thick, opaque fabric with multiple layers.

Securely install curtain rods above the window frame, choosing a rod that complements the nursery decor and supports the curtains' weight. Hang the curtains on rods, ensuring they extend past the window frame to prevent light seeping through the edges.

Test the curtains' effectiveness by closing them during daylight hours and adjusting as needed for naptime and bedtime.

Consider adding a white noise machine or soft music player to enhance the sleep-inducing environment.

By creating a comfortable feeding area and installing blackout curtains, you can create a nurturing and sleep-friendly nursery environment for both you and your baby.

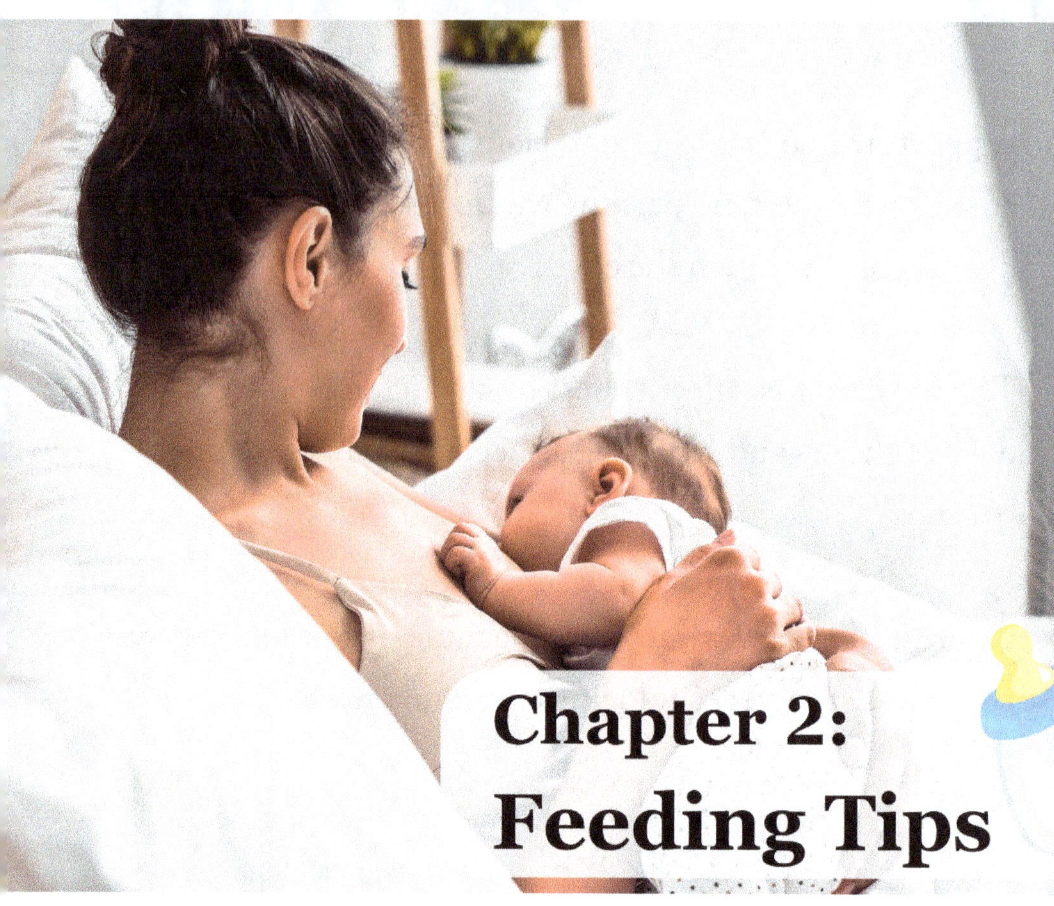

Chapter 2: Feeding Tips

Feeding tips:

Establish a Feeding Schedule

Creating a feeding plan for babies might help them feel more structured and guarantee that they eat enough food all day long. Such as sample below:-

6:00 AM: Feed *(either with formula or breast milk)* after waking up.

8:00 AM: Take a nap

9:30 AM: Take a shower and eat.

11:30 A.M: Take a nap

1:00 PM: Get up and have a meal

3:00 PM: Take a nap

4:30 PM: Get up, eat and drink

6:30 PM: Cluster feeding *(feeding more often to get ready for a longer sleep).*

8:00 PM: Bedtime feeding *(last meal before extended sleep period)*

10:00 PM: Dream feed (**optional;** *give infant a little meal while they're still sleeping to prolong their sleep duration)*

At night:

Feedings infrequently as required (every 3–4 hours) in accordance with the baby's cues.

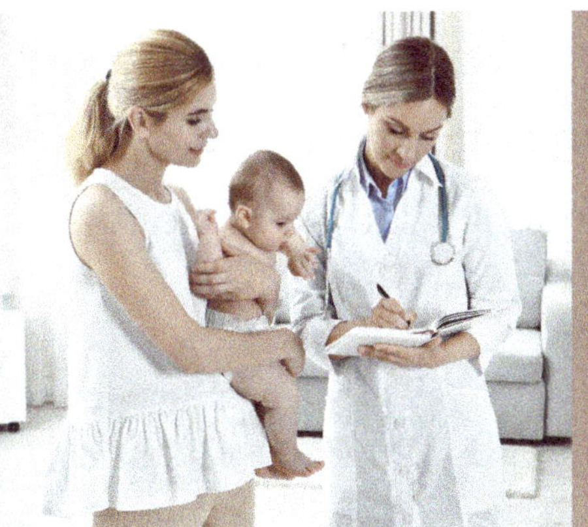

Before establishing a feeding schedule - consult with a pediatrician to ensure it aligns with your baby's nutritional needs and growth requirements.

Understand your baby's hunger cues and respond promptly to avoid overfeeding or underfeeding. Newborns typically feed every 2-3 hours or 8-12 times per day, so feed on demand until they establish a routine.

As your baby grows, aim for a more predictable feeding schedule such as 3-4 hours during the day and longer stretches at night.

Cluster feeding is normal in early evenings, preparing your baby for longer sleep at night. Offer both breast and bottle milk and keep track of feedings using a feeding log.

Be flexible and responsive to your baby's needs, as growth spurts, developmental changes and illness may require adjustments.

Monitor your baby's weight gain regularly and consult your paediatrician if you have concerns about feeding frequency or quantity. As your baby approaches 6 months of age, introduce solid foods alongside breastfeeding or formula feeding, following your paediatrician's recommendations.

Stay hydrated by offering water between feedings once your baby is ready for it, typically around 6 months of age. Remember that every baby is unique, so what works for one may not work for another.

Trust your instincts and seek guidance from healthcare professionals when needed.

Use a Nursing Pillow

It's true that using a nursing cushion might be useful advice for caring for a baby, especially during feeding times. Some advantages and usefulness ideas for utilising it are:

Support: Nursing pillows provide the infant and the carer even more support. They relieve pressure on the caregiver's arms, shoulders and back by raising the infant into a comfortable feeding posture.

Comfort: To provide a pleasant surface for the infant to rest on during feeding sessions, nursing pillows are often made of soft, padded materials.

Appropriate Positioning: The baby's latch and entire feeding experience depend on the nurse or bottle being used properly, which these cushions may assist guarantee.

Bonding: By facilitating greater physical and visual contact, the use of a nursing cushion may improve bonding between the infant and the carer during feeding times.

Versatility: In addition to being used for feeding, nursing pillows may also be used for tummy time and supporting a baby during supervised play.

HINTS FOR MAKING EFFICIENT USE OF A BREASTFEEDING PILLOW:

Before putting the infant on the cushion, make sure it is firmly around your waist. Ensure that it is at a height that is comfortable for feeding.

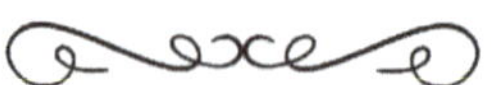

Make sure that the cushion provides enough support for the infant's head, neck and back. *If required,* reposition the cushion to ensure correct alignment.

When utilising the breastfeeding cushion, be mindful of your own posture. During feeding sessions, try to avoid pain by sitting in a chair that is comfortable and provides appropriate back support.

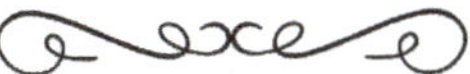

To preserve hygiene, clean the nursing pillow on a regular basis in accordance with the manufacturer's recommendations.

To avoid experiencing pain or discomfort in the nipples, make sure the infant is securely latching onto the breast during nursing. The breastfeeding pillow's support and placement aids may aid in achieving a successful latch.

All things considered, nursing pillows may make feedings more pleasant and comfortable for the infant as well as the carer.

Try Different Nipple Shape Bottles

Selecting the right bottle and nipple shape is important for infant care and feeding. To ensure your baby's comfort and proper feeding, observe their feeding habits and experiment with different shapes, such as - **Standard, Wide-neck, Angled** and **Orthodontic.**

Consider your baby's age and development, as their feeding needs and abilities change over time. For instance, younger infants may prefer a softer, more flexible nipple, while older babies might require a firmer one for better control.

If breastfeeding and supplementing with bottle feeding - consider using nipples designed for breastfed babies, which mimic the natural shape and feel of the breast, making it easier for babies to transition between breast and bottle.

Check for proper fit and flow, ensuring the nipple's flow rate matches your baby's feeding pace and fits securely onto the bottle to prevent leakage and air intake.

Consult a paediatrician or lactation consultant if unsure about the best bottle or nipple shape. They can provide personalised recommendations based on your baby's specific needs and feeding habits.

Be patient and persistent in trying different options until you find the one that works best for your baby.

Burp Baby Properly

Properly burping a baby helps expel air held in their stomach while feeding, decreasing fussiness associated with gas and lowering pain. It's an important element of caring for a child. *See some pointers on how to properly burp a baby:*

Timing: Give your infant a burp halfway through and one more when the meal is complete. This lessens pain both during and after eating and excessive air intake.

Placing your infant upright on your chest or shoulder, use one hand to support their head and neck while giving them a gentle pat or stroke on their back. As an alternative, you might place your infant's face down on your lap, supporting their head and giving their back a little pat or stroke.

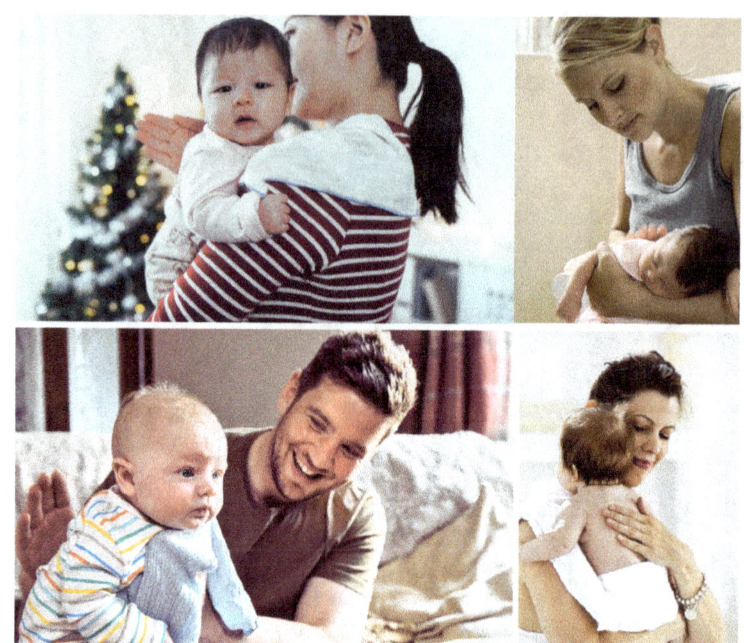

Patting Technique: Firmly yet softly pat your baby's back. Once you determine what pressure and rhythmic motion your baby responds to best, adjust it accordingly. While some newborns react better to soft stroking, others may need patting that is a little stronger.

Remain Calm: Infants are aware of your tension and annoyance. In the event that your infant doesn't burp right away, be calm and patient. Occasionally, it could take several minutes for the burp to appear.

Try Different Positions: Try moving to a different position and trying again if your baby isn't burping after a few minutes in the first one. A baby may have a preference for a certain posture.

Refrain from overfeeding your infant as this may cause pain and increased air swallowing. Keep an eye out for signs that indicate your baby is full, such as turning away from the breast or bottle, shutting their lips, or losing interest in eating.

Tips for Bottle-Feeding: To reduce air intake, make sure the nipple is full of milk while you're bottle-feeding. Tilt

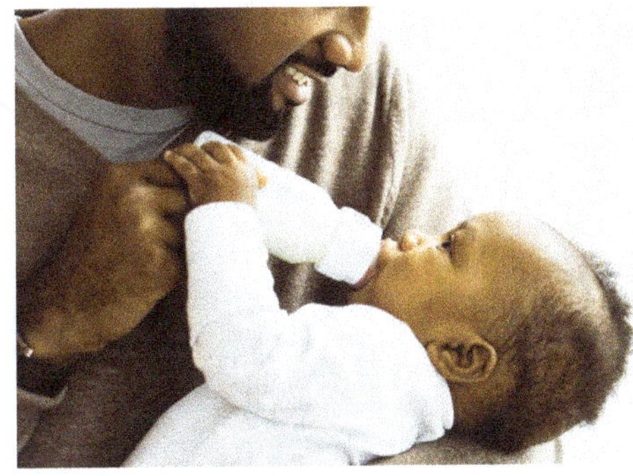

the bottle so that air rises to the top and the milk fills the nipple fully.

Burping Frequency: If a baby is formula-fed or has a tendency to swallow air, they may need more frequent burping than other newborns. Observe your baby's indications and modify your burping technique as necessary.

Pump and Store Breastmilk

Storage Recommendations: Depending on when you want to use it - breast milk may be kept at room temperature, in the refrigerator or frozen:-

* **At room temperature** (77°F or 25°C), breast milk may be kept for up to **4** hours without risk.

* **Refrigerator:** Breast milk may be safely kept for up to **4–8** days at **32–39°F (0–4°C)**.

* Breast milk may be securely kept in a freezer section of a refrigerator (**at 5°F or -15°C**) for up to **2** weeks.

* Breast milk may be securely kept in a freezer with a separate door at **0°F or -18°C** for up to **6–12** months.

When it's time to utilise the breast milk that has been frozen, defrost it by either putting the container in the refrigerator for the whole night or by slowly heating it in a bowl of warm water.

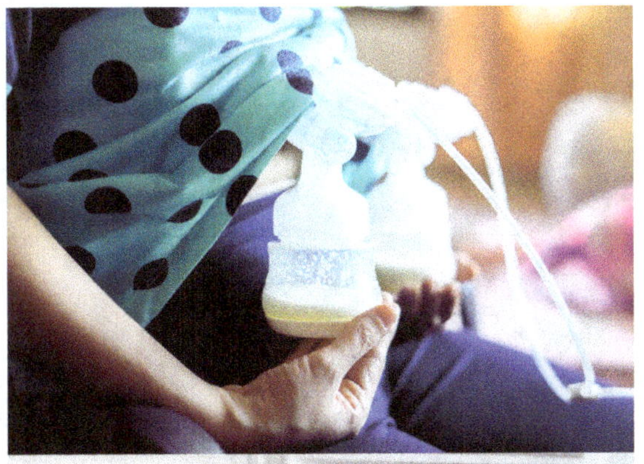

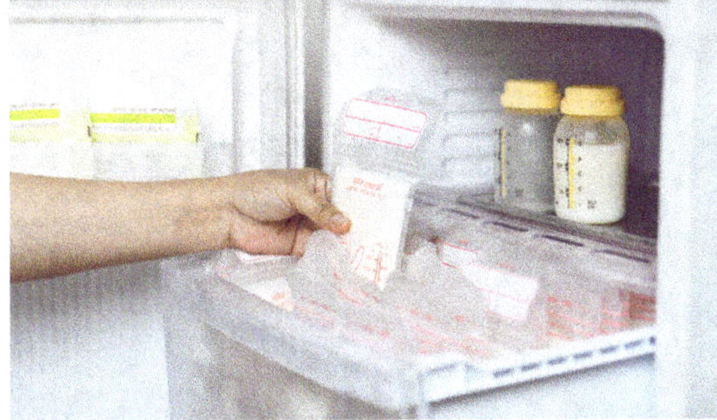

Breast milk pumping is a common practice for mothers who want to continue breastfeeding while feeding their baby when they're not physically present.

To pump and store breast milk, you need the right equipment, such as a double electric pump and storage bottles or bags specifically designed for breast milk storage.

Clean and sanitize your equipment before starting. Choose a comfortable spot to pump without interruptions. Prepare yourself by gently massage your breasts or applying a warm compress to stimulate milk flow. Position the breast shield properly to ensure a good seal around your nipple.

Start pumping by starting with a low suction setting and gradually increasing the suction strength until you find a comfortable level. Pump for 15-20 minutes per session or until your breasts feel empty. Store the breast milk in storage bottles or bags, labeling each container with the date the milk was expressed.

Breast milk should never be microwaved as it might lose important nutrients and produce hot patches that could burn your baby's mouth.

Clean Up: As directed by the manufacturer, be sure to thoroughly clean and sanitise your breast pump and all of its components once you've completed pumping.

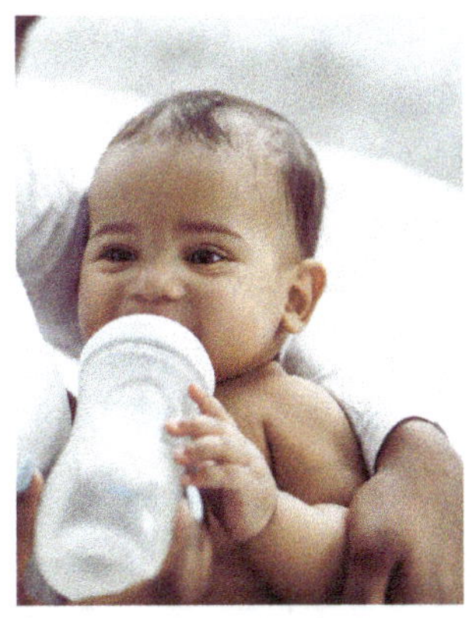

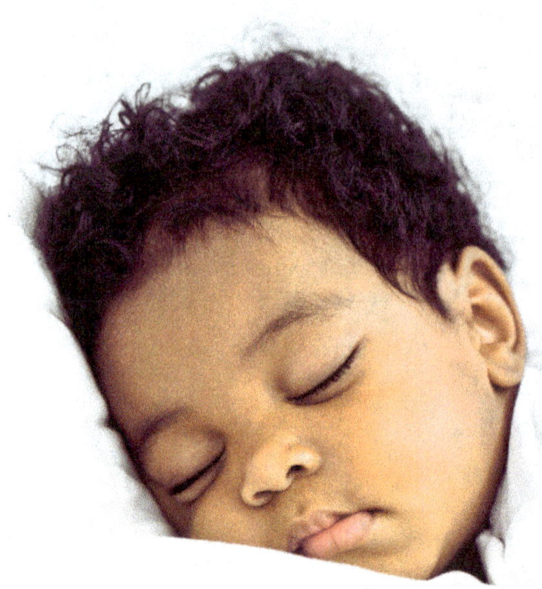

Chapter 3: Sleeping Hac

Sleeping Hacks:

Swaddle Baby And Use White Noise to Aid Better Sleep

It's true that swaddling newborns and playing white noise are common ways to improve their quality of sleep.

Here's why they function as well as some further advice:

Swaddling: Swaddling gives a newborn a feeling of security and comfort by simulating the warm, protective environment of the womb. Moreover, it inhibits the startle reaction, which awakens infants. To lower the risk of Sudden Infant Death Syndrome **(SIDS)**, always lay the baby to sleep on their back after swaddling and make sure the blanket is snug but not too tight.

White Noise: White noise generators or applications provide a continuous, calming sound that resembles what foetuses perceive. This soothing tone may help block out other sounds that might rouse the infant from sleep and provide a peaceful sleeping environment.

Additional Advice: Create a Bedtime Routine

Regular night time routine: Create a regular night time schedule that include relaxing activities such as reading a bedtime tale, taking a warm bath and receiving a light massage. The infant receives this pattern as a cue to go to sleep.

Establish a sleep-friendly atmosphere by making sure the baby's room is calm, dark and at a suitable temperature. To reduce light, use blackout curtains and think about getting a cosy mattress or other sleeping surface.

Keep an eye out for your baby's cues: Look for symptoms of fatigue, such as wiping of the eyes, yawning or fussiness. When a baby is sleepy but not asleep, putting them to bed or for a nap might help them learn how to self-soothe and go asleep on their own.

Safe sleep practices: When a baby goes to sleep, they should always do so on their back on a firm mattress free of any toys, blankets or pillows that might suffocate them. Make sure the infant is wearing airy, light clothes to prevent overheating.

Since each infant is unique - what works for one may not work for another, so exercise patience and flexibility. Have patience and be open to experimenting with various tactics until you figure out what suits your infant the best.

Remember that babies have erratic sleep cycles and could wake up often to feed, it's important to be adaptable and sensitive to their demands while establishing sound sleeping habits.

Use a Nightlight for Middle-of-the-Night Diaper Changes and Encourage Naps Throughout the Day.

Using a nightlight for middle-of-the-night diaper changes is a beneficial strategy for infant care, as it creates a gentle, soothing environment that doesn't disturb the baby too much.

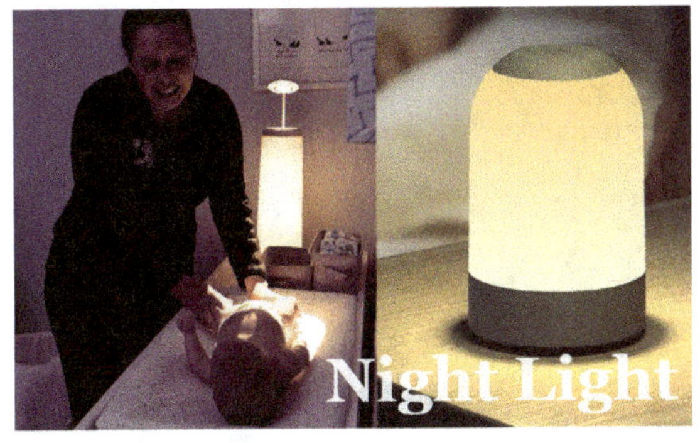

To effectively use a nightlight, choose a soft, warm glow such as LED nightlights and position it strategically near the changing table or nursery. Maintain a calm environment during diaper changes to help the baby transition back to sleep.

Maintain a consistent night time routine to signal to the baby that it's time for sleep. Incorporate the nightlight into this routine to associate it with bedtime.

Encouraging naps throughout the day is also essential for infant care, as babies need plenty of rest to support their growth and development. To promote daytime naps, create a comfortable sleep environment, establish a regular nap schedule based on your baby's natural sleep patterns and pay attention to sleep cues like rubbing their eyes, yawning or becoming fussy.

Be flexible and responsive to your baby's individual sleep needs, as some days may require more or longer naps than others.

By incorporating these strategies into your infant care routine, you can ensure your baby gets the rest they need to thrive and grow.

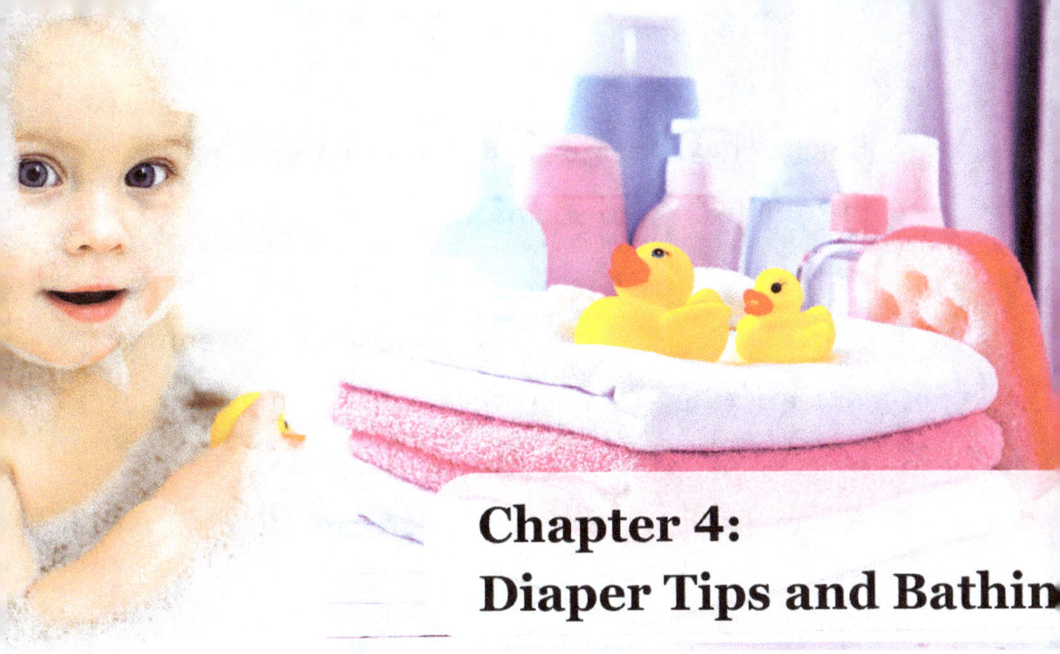

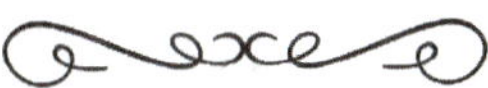

Chapter 4:
Diaper Tips and Bathin

Diaper Tips and Bathing:

Diapering is a crucial aspect of a baby's life and it's important to choose the right diapers for your baby's size and weight.

Create a designated changing station with necessary supplies like diapers, wipes, diaper rash cream and a changing pad.

❖ Regularly check diapers, especially after feedings or naps to prevent soiled diapers.

- ❖ Ensure the diaper fits snugly but not too tight to prevent leaks or discomfort.

- ❖ Prevent diaper rash by changing diapers promptly and applying a thin layer of cream during changes.

- ❖ Allow your baby to go diaper-free for short periods to air out their skin.

- ❖ Consider using overnight diapers for longer dryness and reduced disturbances during sleep.

Bathing Tips:

To bathe a newborn, start every 2-3 days until the umbilical cord stump falls off, then 2-3 times per week.

- ❖ Ensure the room is warm and draft-free with water temperature around 37°C (98.6°F).

- ❖ Gather necessary supplies, such as mild baby soap, a soft washcloth, towel, clean clothes and bath toys.

❖ Support your baby by keeping one hand on their head and neck.

❖ Use a mild soap and gently wash their body, paying attention to creases, folds and diaper area.

❖ Pat dry with a soft towel, paying extra attention to skin folds.

❖ Apply gentle baby lotion or oil to keep their skin moisturised, especially in dry climates or winter months.

Choosing the Right Diaper Brand and Use a Diaper Pail for Odour Control

Choosing the Correct Diaper Brand:

Take Your Baby's Sensitivity Into Account - Diapers should be mild and hypoallergenic since some newborns may have sensitive skin.

Absorbency: To keep your baby dry and comfortable for extended periods of time, choose for diapers with a high absorbency.

Fit: To stop leaks, diapers should fit tightly around the waist and legs. Diapers made especially for babies are available from several companies.

Material: To lower your chance of diaper rash and discomfort, use breathable diapers.

Reviews and Advice: To get knowledge about the performance of various nappy brands, ask other parents for advice or read internet reviews.

Trial and Error: Since each baby is different, it might take some experimenting to determine which brand is best for your child.

Utilising a Diaper Pail to Manage Odour:

Selecting the Proper Diaper Pail Choose a diaper pail made especially to hold scents.

Certain pails are equipped with extra features like antibacterial protection and hands-free functionality.

Diaper Proper Disposal: Before putting diapers in the diaper pail, make sure they are firmly sealed.

Frequent Emptying: To avoid odours building up, empty the diaper pail on a frequent basis. Emptying the diaper on a daily basis is advised, particularly for newborns and babies who could go through many diapers in a day.

Odour Neutralizers: You may choose to use scented bags or deodorising discs, which are odour-neutralising items made specifically for diaper pails.

Cleaning: To avoid bacteria growth and residual smells, wash the diaper pail on a regular basis using a mild soap and water.

Location: To reduce odours, place the diaper pail in a well-ventilated spot away from strong sunlight and busy streets.

Choosing the ideal diaper brand and using diaper pail practices correctly can help you keep your kid comfortable and your house odour-free during diaper changes.

Bathe Baby Using Warm Water and Bath Thermometer for Safety.

Giving a newborn or infant a bath may be a wonderful way for parents and children to spend quality time together.

Here are some pointers to guarantee comfort and safety:

Assemble Supplies: Before beginning the bath, place all required materials at your fingertips. This contains a clean diaper, clean clothing, a soft washcloth, a towel and any other necessities for bathing.

Select the Ideal Time: Opt for a moment when your infant isn't very fatigued or hungry. Bathing a baby before going to sleep is something that many parents believe helps create a peaceful habit.

Set the Room Temperature: To keep your infant from being cold during the bath, make sure the room is appropriately warm, between 75°F and 80°F (24°C and 27°C).

Get the bathroom ready: Pour warm water into a sanitised baby tub or sink. Make sure the water temperature is between 90°F and 100°F (32°C and 38°C) by using a bath thermometer. To make sure the water isn't excessively hot, feel the temperature with your wrist or elbow.

Carefully take off your baby's clothes, making sure they're cosy and out of the way of drafts. Till you're ready to submerge them in the water - keep them covered in a towel.

Support Baby's Head: Support your infant's head and neck with one hand while keeping a firm grip on them. Never, ever leave your infant alone in the bathtub—not even for a split second.

Wash Gently: To gently clean your baby's body, use a gentle washcloth and mild baby soap. Beginning with their face, proceed to their body and conclude with their posterior. Particular care should be paid to folds and wrinkles where moisture and grime might collect.

Rinse Well: Gently rinse the soap off of your baby's skin using a cup or your hand. Verify that there is no soap residue behind.

Dry and Dress: After removing your child from the bathtub, gently pat them dry with a warm towel. Pay close attention to drying any wrinkles and the space between their fingers and toes. Put on a new nappy and clean clothing for your child.

After the bath, you may, *if necessary,* apply a little baby lotion or moisturiser. If your baby's nails are long, trim them and make sure they are content and at ease.

Savour Time Spent Together: Giving your child a bath may be a really special time spent together. To deepen your bond with your infant, sing or converse with them while they're bathing.

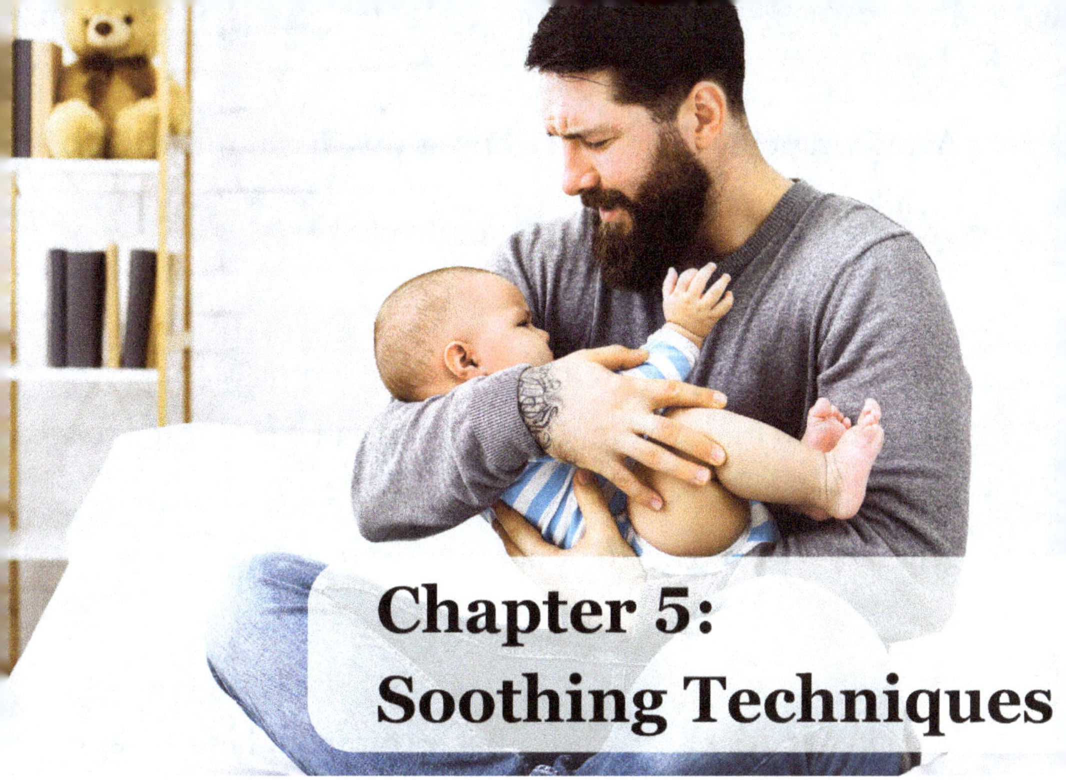

Chapter 5: Soothing Techniques

Soothing Techniques:

Taking care of a newborn or baby can be both rewarding and challenging.

Swaddling: Your baby will feel more at ease and comfortable if you wrap them up tightly in a nice blanket.

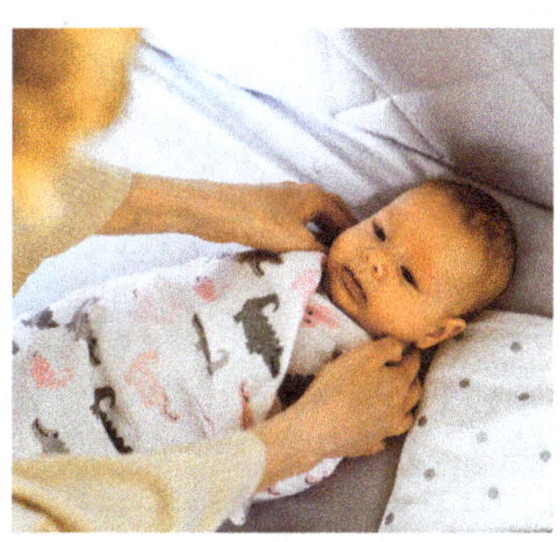

Avoid wrapping them too tightly as this may impede their breathing or mobility.

White noise: Because it may replicate the noises they experienced in the womb, white noise can be soothing to a lot of newborns. This might be a fan, a white noise generator or even a rain or ocean wave recording.

Swaying or Rocking Gently: Babies often find movement to be calming. You may take them for a leisurely stroll in a pram or carrier, rock them in your arms or use a baby swing or rocker.

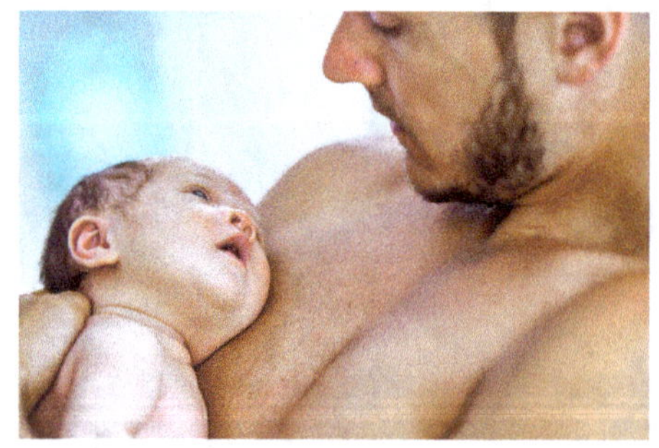

Skin-to-Skin Contact: Your baby's body temperature, heart rate and respiration may all be regulated by holding them close to your chest. Also, it may foster a sense of security and camaraderie.

Sucking: A baby's instinctive need to suck may help soothe them. If you're nursing, encourage them to nurse or offer them your finger as a dummy.

Massage: You may help your baby relax and get better sleep by giving them a gentle massage on their arms, legs and back. Pay 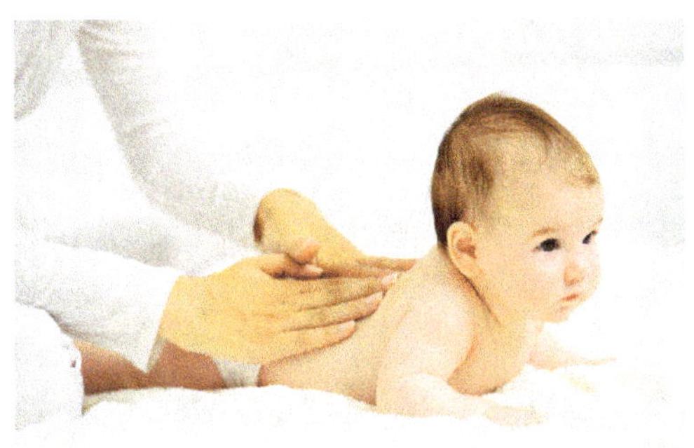 attention to your baby's instincts and move in gentle, circular movements.

Warm Bath: A warm bath may help parents and newborns relax. When giving your infant a bath, make sure the water is at a safe temperature and support their head and neck.

Lullabies or Gentle Music: Your infant might feel more at ease in an environment that is quiet and peaceful. Playing soft music or singing together may help strengthen relationships.

 Newborns may find bright lights to be too much to handle. Using a nightlight or lowering the lights might help your baby feel more at ease, particularly while feedings or changing diapers late at night.

Comfort Objects: A nice blanket, plush animal or other soft item may provide solace to some newborns. Verify that your infant can safely use these things and stay away from anything that has little pieces that might be a choking danger.

Using A Baby Swing or Rocker

You as a parent may enjoy some hands-free time while your baby is calmed down by using a baby swing or chair. Follow these guide to help you use a baby swing or rocker in a safe and efficient manner:

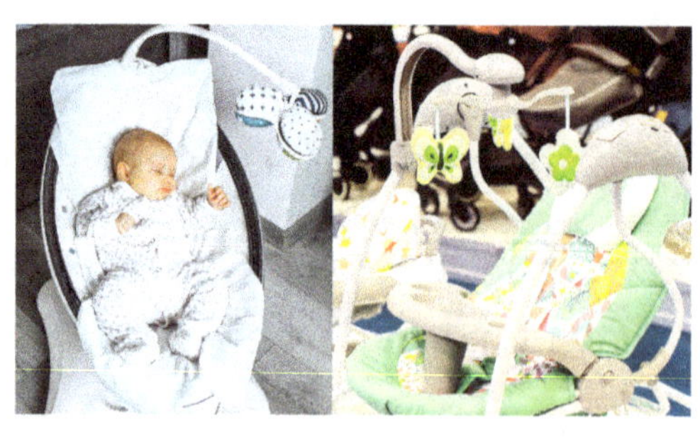

Select the ideal rocker or swing for your baby: There are various varieties of rockers and swings for babies, including ones that rocked side to side or back and forth.

Make sure it satisfies safety regulations and choose one that is appropriate for your baby's weight and size.

Go over the directions: Make sure you understand how to build and operate the swing or rocker properly by carefully reading the manufacturer's instructions before using it.

Observe weight restrictions, safety measures and suggested use instructions.

Make sure the swing or rocker is positioned correctly by setting it on a level, sturdy platform and keeping it clear of any obstructions like cables, drapes or other furniture.

To keep your infant safely fastened, always use the included harness or safety straps.

Start with low speed settings: On the swing or rocker, start with the lowest speed setting and observe your baby's reaction. While some infants could love a quicker rate, others might prefer a soft, calm rocking motion.

Watch over your child: If your child is too small or unable to hold their head and neck on their own, you should never leave them in a swing or rocker alone. Always be on the lookout for them, and be prepared to step in if needed.

Use them Sparingly: Rockers and swings may be useful for calming your infant, but you should only use them sparingly. It's crucial that your infant has chances for exercise and socialisation with carers, so try not to leave them in the swing or rocker for long amounts of time.

Use as a calming tool: When your baby is unhappy or in need of comforting, use the swing or rocker into your soothing routine, such as before bedtime or naptime. For best results, use it with additional calming methods like white noise, swaddling or soft rocking.

Change from the swing or rocker: As your child becomes older and more mature, you may need to gently move them from these comfortable places to alternative calming activities like holding them close, playing independently or nursing.

Chapter 6: Health and Safety

Keep Baby's Room at the Right Temperature

Since newborns and infants are more susceptible to temperature extremes than adults, it is imperative that you keep your baby's room at the proper temperature for their health and safety.

Some pointers in keeping your surroundings cosy and secure:

Recommended Room Temperature: A baby's room should be between 68°F and 72°F (**20°C and 22.2°C**). For most newborns, this range is safe and pleasant.

Use a Thermometer: Continually check the temperature in your baby's room by placing a trustworthy thermometer there. Accurate measurements may be obtained with ease of reading using digital thermometers.

Prevent Overheating: Your baby may feel uncomfortable and there's a higher chance of **SIDS** if they become too hot. Steer clear of utilising bulky blankets or overdressing your infant. Wear light clothes that are suitable for the room temperature while dressing your infant.

Use a Fan: To keep the space from becoming too stuffy, you may use a portable or ceiling fan to assist move air about. Make sure your infant cannot reach the fan and that it is not blowing straight into their face.

Maintain Good Ventilation: Keeping a healthy indoor environment requires enough ventilation. To let in fresh air, open windows or doors, but make sure there are no drafts straight onto your baby's cot.

Observe for Climatic or Overheating Signs: To tell whether your infant is too hot or too cold, pay attention to their indications. Sweating, flushed cheeks, fast breathing and irritation are symptoms of being overheated. Shivering, fussiness, chilly hands and feet are indicators of extreme cold.

Modify Bedding: Make use of breathable, light-weight blankets and sheets made of cotton. Steer clear of bulky blankets or comforters that might trap heat. To prevent suffocation, use a wearable blanket or sleep sack to keep your infant warm.

Avoid Heat Sources: Keep your infant's cot out of the direct sunshine, heaters and radiators since they may rapidly raise the room's temperature and produce hot spots.

Consider/Get a Room Thermometer with Alarm: Some infant monitors have room thermometers built in that will notify you if the temperature deviates from the recommended range. More peace of mind may result from this, particularly at night.

Be Consistent: To assist your baby in developing a good sleep schedule, make an effort to keep the temperature of your room at the same level throughout the day and at night.

You can make sure that your baby's room stays at the ideal temperature for their health and safety by following these instructions.

Use a Humidifier for Congestion

When a newborn or baby has congestion, using a humidifier may assist relieve their pain and encourage improved breathing.

See how to operate a humidifier in a safe and efficient manner:

Selecting the Correct Type of Humidifier: **Warm mist** and **Cool mist** humidifiers are the two basic varieties. Cool mist humidifiers are often advised for infants due to the fact that they reduce the chance of burns by not heating the water.

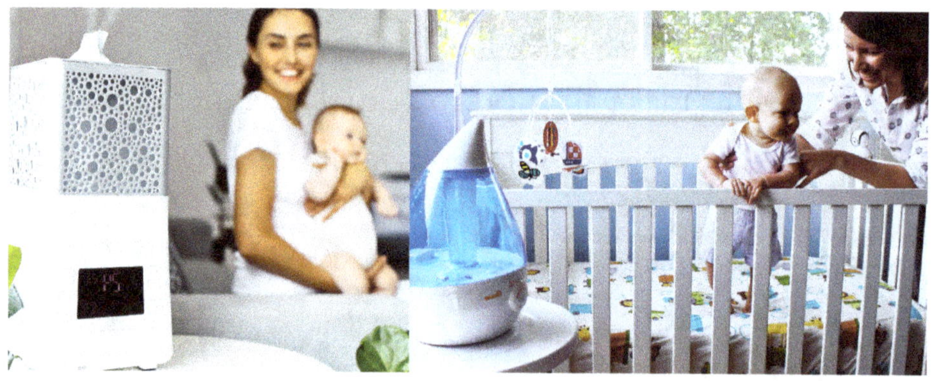

Keep It Clean: Make sure there is no bacteria or mould growth on the humidifier. Observe the maintenance and cleaning guidelines provided by the manufacturer. To stop dangerous germs from growing, clean the unit and replace the water on a regular basis.

Use Purified or Distilled Water: Using purified or distilled water in the humidifier may aid in preventing the airborne dissemination of pollutants and minerals that might endanger the developing respiratory system of your child.

Place it Safely: To reduce the possibility of unintentional spills or leaks, place the humidifier a safe distance away from the baby's bed or cot. It needs to be set up on a sturdy surface that is difficult to topple.

Monitor Humidity Levels: Pay attention to the room's humidity levels. For newborns, the optimal humidity range is **30%** to **50%.** While too little humidity might worsen respiratory problems and congestion, too much humidity can promote the formation of mould.

Use as directed: To use the humidifier, according to the manufacturer's operating manual. Certain models could include mist output and humidity settings that can be changed. If your infant is uncomfortable, start with a lower setting and make adjustments as necessary.

Think About Using Saline Drops: To assist your baby's nasal passages clear out, you may use saline nasal drops or saline spray in addition to a humidifier. For information on proper dose and use, speak with your paediatrician.

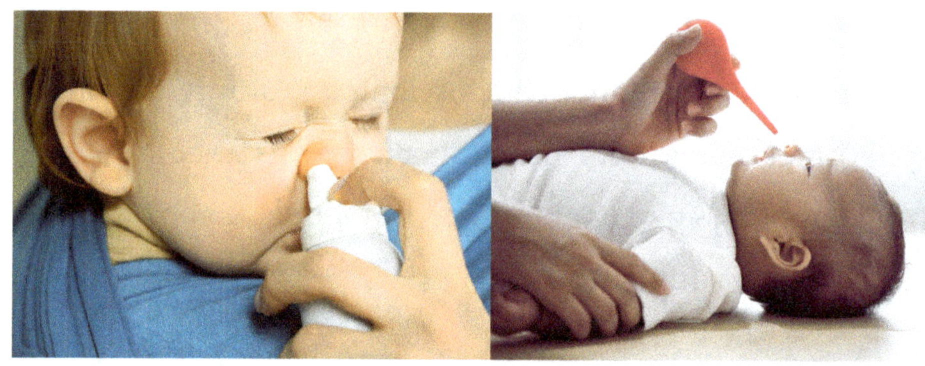

Keep watch for Improvement or Worsening: Although a humidifier may help reduce congestion, it's important to keep a careful eye on your baby's symptoms. See your paediatrician right once if you see any indications of increased congestion, breathing difficulties or other worrisome symptoms.

Do note that treating congestion in newborns and babies involves more than simply using a humidifier. Maintaining a clean environment for your infant and practising proper hygiene, such regular handwashing, are also important to reducing the risk of respiratory infections.

Please don't hesitate to see your paediatrician if you have any questions about the usage of a humidifier or your baby's health.

Install Outlet Covers and Baby Gates

Installing Outlet Covers:

The market offers a wide range of outlet cover kinds. Select those that are made with kid safety in mind.

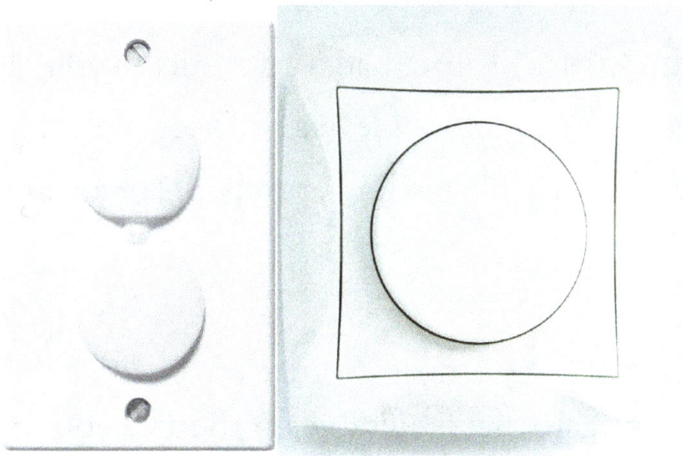

Turn off Power: To reduce the chance of electric shock, turn off the main circuit breaker's power to the outlets you'll be working on before putting outlet covers.

Remove Any Existing Covers: If there are any outlet covers, use a screwdriver to gently remove them.

Install Outlet Covers: Make sure the outlet covers fit tightly in the sockets by inserting them there. While some outlet covers may be installed without screws, others need to be plugged into the sockets.

Test: After installation, make sure that all outlet covers are firmly in place and difficult for kids to remove.

Cover All Outlets: Ensure that every outlet in your house, including the ones at lower levels and accessible to young children who are still crawling or walking, is covered.

How to Install Baby Gates:

Select a baby gate that is suitable for the area you want to keep open. Hardware-mounted gates and pressure mounted gates are two of the several varieties that are available.

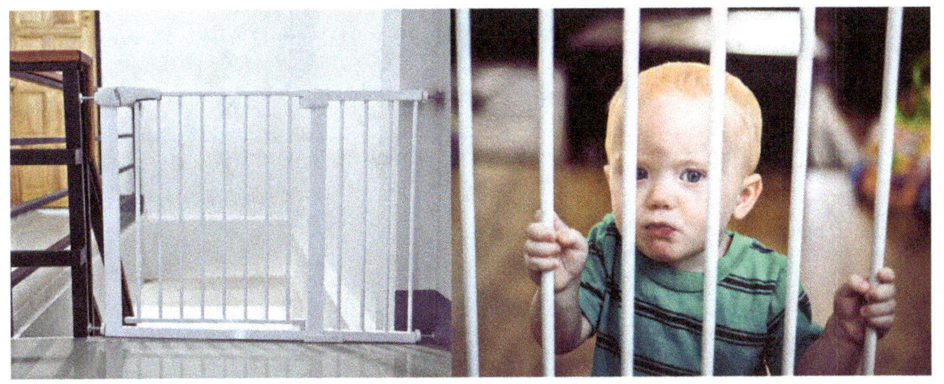

Measure the Space: To find the width of the entryway or aperture where you want to put the gate, use a tape measure.

Installing a Pressure-Mounted Gate is as easy as positioning it in the doorway or opening and adjusting the tension to lock it in place. Verify that the gate is sturdy and level.

Install Hardware-Mounted Gate: Mark the location of the gate brackets on the wall or door frame with a pencil for hardware-mounted gates. Drill pilot holes before firmly screwing the brackets into position. As directed by the manufacturer - attach the gate to the brackets.

Test the Gate: After installation, make sure the gate locks firmly and opens and shuts smoothly.

Look for Safety Hazards: Verify that your youngster won't be put in danger by any gaps or sharp edges. Make sure the gate is high enough to discourage anyone from climbing over it.

Watch over: Although they act as a barrier, baby gates cannot take the place of parental monitoring. Always be aware of your child's whereabouts, particularly if they are close to the gate.

By adding outlet covers and baby gates, you can successfully childproof your house and provide your newborn or infant a safer environment.

Keep Poisonous Substances Out of Reach

It is essential for the protection and wellbeing of newborns and babies to keep toxic materials out of reach.

Some crucial pointers to guarantee their safety are:

Lock up Chemicals and Medications: Keep any cleaning supplies, vitamins, medicines and chemicals for the home secured in cupboards or high shelves out of children's reach. When not in use, make sure they are well closed.

Install childproof locks on cabinets and drawers that contain dangerous materials to make them childproof. These locks help keep inquisitive babies away from potentially dangerous objects.

Be Aware of Plants: If consumed - several indoor and outdoor plants may be harmful. Keep poisonous plants out of your child's reach and be mindful of any plants in your surroundings or at home that can be dangerous.

Safe Storage of Personal Care goods: Chemicals that might be dangerous can be found in goods like cosmetics, fragrances and personal care items. Keep them securely out of children's reach; cabinets with childproof locks are ideal.

Tight-fitting lids on lockable garbage containers are a good way to dispose of hazardous objects including batteries, home cleansers and pharmaceuticals. Never put these things in plain sight in containers where kids may get them.

Label Hazardous Items Properly: Make sure that any containers containing potentially harmful materials have labels that are simple to read and that are clearly visible.

- This covers prescription drugs, household cleaners and any other potentially dangerous substances.

Educate Carers: Share with grandparents, babysitters and other carers the significance of keeping toxic materials out of children's reach. Give precise instructions on how to handle and where to keep these objects.

Exercise Caution When Using Pest Control Products: Make sure to store pest control products safely and use them in accordance with the manufacturer's directions whether you use them inside or outside of your house.

Whenever feasible, try to choose non-toxic substitutes, particularly in places where kids may easily reach them.

Check Your house Frequently for risks: Make sure to regularly examine your house to find and fix any possible risks. This entails looking for anything that might endanger your kid, such as loose or leaky containers, outdated prescriptions and other things.

Emergency Preparedness: Become familiar with what to do in the event of an unintentional poisoning. Know the warning signs and symptoms of poisoning and have the Poison Control Center's emergency contact information at hand.

Learn CPR for Infants

Anyone who spends time with newborns, including parents and carers, should become proficient in baby CPR *(cardiopulmonary resuscitation)*. In an emergency when a baby's breathing or heartbeat has stopped, CPR may save lives.

The following is a detailed tutorial on how to administer CPR to a baby:

Step 1: Evaluate the circumstances

To ensure safety, evaluate the baby and the surroundings before beginning CPR. CPR is required if the baby is unresponsive or not breathing at all.

Step 2: Make a Help Request

If you're by yourself, give yourself CPR for around 20 minutes before calling 911 for help. While you begin CPR, ask everyone else in the room to phone emergency services right away.

Step 3: Clear the Airway

The baby should be placed on their back on a solid surface. To clear their airway, tilt their head back a little and elevate their chin.

Step 4: Examine Your Breath

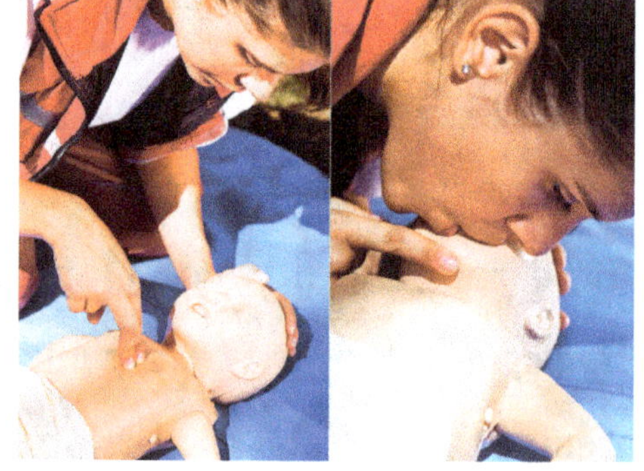

Watch, hear and feel your breathing. Keep an eye out for a rise in your chest, listen for breath noises and feel your cheek for breath. Start CPR if the baby is not breathing regularly.

Step 5: Compress your chest.

Apply light compressions to the chest using two fingers, preferably the middle and ring fingers. Put your fingers in the baby's chest in the middle, slightly below the nipple line.

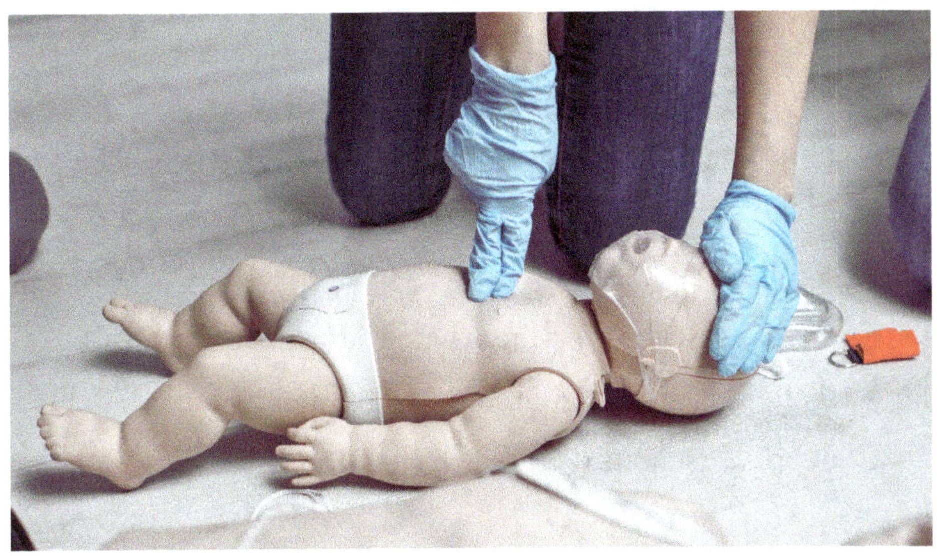

Press the chest down to a depth of about 1.5 inches, using 100–120 compressions each minute. A complete recoil of the chest is allowed in between compressions.

Step 6: Inhale life-saving air

Deliver two rescue breaths after thirty compressions. Keep the head tilted and chin up, cover the baby's mouth and nose with your mouth and blow air for a few seconds at a time while keeping an eye out for a rise in the chest.

Step 7: Carry out again

Repeat cycles of two rescue breaths followed by 30 chest compressions until assistance comes or the baby begins breathing on its own.

Summary:

- Regularly check respiration and responsiveness.
- Make sure you're breathing and compressing the right way.
- Save CPR for checking the patient's breathing alone.
- If there is an automated external defibrillator (AED) nearby, use it and adhere to its instructions.

It's imperative that you enrol in a CPR training course that covers baby CPR, since practical experience and guidance from a certified teacher will boost your self-assurance and competence in delivering CPR.

Furthermore, while taking care of newborns, always put safety first and have emergency numbers on hand.

Chapter 7: Travelling with Baby

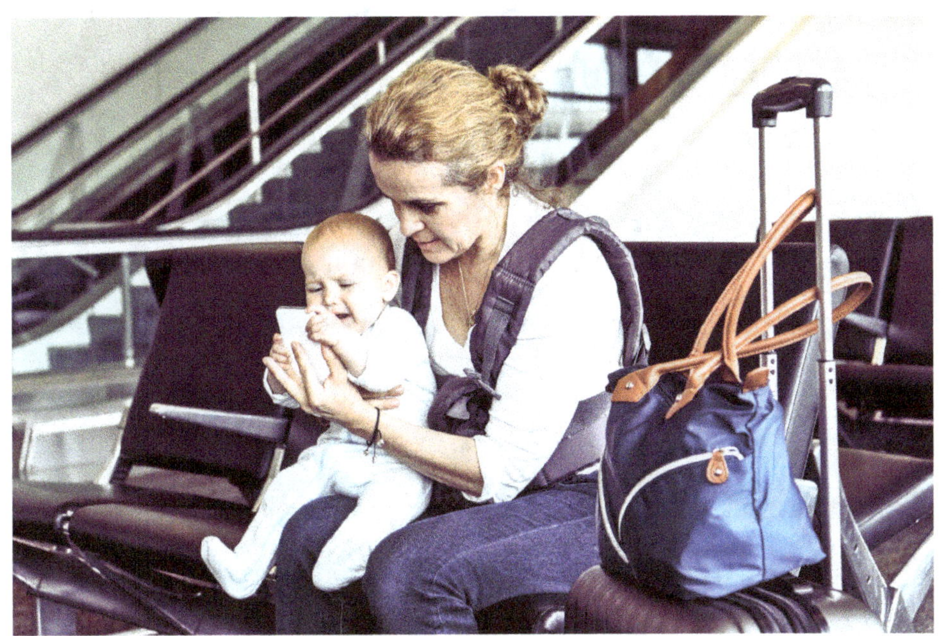

Pack a Diaper Bag Essentials Kit and Use a Portable Changing Pad.

It's important to be well-prepared for every eventuality while travelling with a newborn. Bringing along a portable change mat and an essentials pack for your diaper bag will help ensure a lot easier travel.

Here's how to maximise the use of a portable changing mat and arrange your diaper bag basics kit:

Essentials for a Diaper Bag Kit

Diapers: Bring enough diapers for the number of times a day you usually need them, plus a few extras in case of emergencies.

Wipes: For quick cleanups, always have a travel-sized box of baby wipes on hand. For convenience, individually wrapped wipes are another option.

Diaper Rash Cream: To relieve your baby's skin, provide a little tube or travel-sized container of diaper rash cream.

Changing Pad: If your diaper bag doesn't include a built-in changing pad, you may want to choose a foldable or portable one. When changing diapers, these pads provide a hygienic and cosy surface, particularly if you're on the move.

Extra clothing: If your baby spills or has an accident, make sure they have at least one change of clothing. If it's going to be cool outside, pack a jumper, a cap and socks.

Bring a couple disposable plastic bags with you in case your clothes and diapers become filthy. They lessen spills and help keep odours contained in your diaper bag.

Hand Sanitizer: For easy cleanups before and after diaper changes, include a travel-sized bottle of hand sanitizer in your diaper bag.

Burp Cloths or Bibs: To keep their clothing clean, carry a few burp cloths or bibs if your kid has a tendency to spit up.

Feeding Supplies: Pack bottles, formula and an insulated bag or bottle warmer to keep the bottles warm if you're bottle-feeding. Add nursing pads and, *if preferred,* a nursing cover for nursing.

Toys or Pacifiers: Pack a few little toys or pacifiers to assist keep your baby occupied and relaxed while changing diapers or travelling.

Transportable Changing Pad:
When you need to change your baby's diaper in a public toilet or another unhygienic setting, a portable changing mat is an absolute must.

Seek for a changing mat that is both easily cleaned and waterproof. To hold diapers, wipes and other necessities, some pads even include pockets or sections.

Fold the changing mat and store it in your diaper bag for convenient access while not in use.

Using a portable changing mat and keeping an adequately supplied diaper bag essentials kit can help you be more equipped to deal with last-minute scenarios and diaper changes while travelling with your infant.

Consider a Bassinet Attachment for Strollers

A bassinet attachment may come in rather handy while travelling with a baby, particularly if you want to use a pram. It can benefit both you and your child.

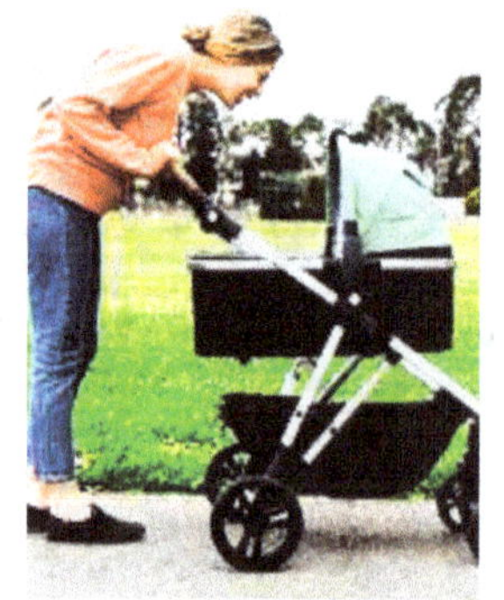

The following justifies giving a bassinet attachment for your pram considerable thought:

Comfort: Your infant may sleep comfortably in a bassinet while you're on the road. Because it provides a level surface, it is advised for newborns and early babies as it supports the development of their neck and spine.

Safety: A bassinet offers a secure and pleasant resting environment for your baby, lowering the danger of positional asphyxiation. This is in contrast to infant car seats, which are useful for transport but not the best for extended periods of sleep because of their inclined posture.

Convenience: Easily attachable and removable bassinet accessories from the stroller frame provide smooth transitions between walking and sleeping. This implies that you may take your dozing child from the pram to your house or place of lodging without waking them up.

Longevity: Unlike other infant car seats, which babies outgrow fast, many bassinet attachments are appropriate for newborns and infants up to a certain weight or age.

Interaction: By placing your infant at a stroller's height, a bassinet attachment helps you and your child develop a closer link and increase communication.

Ventilation: Compared to car seats or stroller seats, bassinets usually provide greater ventilation, which may assist control your baby's temperature and avoid overheating.

Versatility: Some bassinet attachments may be used as stand-alone sleepers or in conjunction with strollers, giving them adaptable travel alternatives.

Think about things like stroller model compatibility, safety features, portability and convenience of use when selecting a bassinet attachment. Also, to guarantee your baby's safety while travelling - always adhere to the manufacturer's instructions and suggestions for safe sleeping techniques.

Use a Car Seat Mirror for Monitoring Baby

Safety and close supervision are important while travelling with a baby, particularly in an automobile. One useful item for seeing your infant while driving is a car seat mirror.

Correct Installation: Verify that the vehicle seat mirror is mounted firmly and in the right place. The majority of mirrors use suction cups or adjustable straps to fasten to the rear windscreen or headrest of the back seat. For correct installation, adhere to the manufacturer's instructions.

Positioning: Set up the mirror so you can see your child's face clearly while driving. It needs to be positioned such that you can easily see the baby's image in your rearview mirror.

Check the View: Make sure you can see your infant well in the mirror before you start driving. Examine many perspectives to determine the ideal arrangement.

Frequent glances: Check on your infant by glancing in the mirror from time to time while you're driving. But keep in mind that you should keep your eyes on the road.

Avoid Distractions: Keeping an eye on your infant is important, but don't let it divert you from safe driving. Instead, try not to become too hooked on the mirror.

To check on your infant without taking your eyes off the road for too long, make brief, discrete glances.

Adjust as Necessary: Stop and readjust the mirror if you detect any movement or shifting while driving. Keeping an unobstructed view of your infant is vital.

Though visual monitoring is provided by a car seat mirror, you should think about employing additional baby monitoring devices, such as rear-facing camera systems in your car or baby monitors, *if they are available.* These may provide additional comfort, particularly on extended trips.

When Not in Use - Take Out the Car Seat Mirror: Take out the car seat mirror from the car when you're not taking your infant along. This keeps it from becoming dangerous in the case of an accident or abrupt pauses.

Plan for Breastfeeding or Formula Feeding on the Go

Whether you're travelling by car, airline or any other kind of conveyance, you need to prepare ahead to make sure your baby's feeding requirements are satisfied.

Here's a strategy for on-the-go formula and nursing feedings:

BreastFeeding

Bring the necessities:

Nursing cover: When nursing in public, a lightweight nursing cover offers privacy.

Extra nursing pads: To remain dry, carry extra nursing pads since leaks might occur.

Breast pump (*optional*)**:** A portable breast pump might come in helpful for expressing milk if you're going to be away from your infant for a long time.

Schedule Meals Breaks: Plan frequent pauses where you can comfortably nurse your child if you're driving.
Be mindful of the airline's nursing restrictions if you're travelling by air. Breastfeeding is permitted on most airlines during flights.

Recognise Your Rights: Learn about the local regulations pertaining to breastfeeding in public so you may legally and comfortably nurse your baby wherever you go.

Keep Yourself Hydrated and Fed: In order to sustain your energy levels and milk production, don't forget to consume healthy snacks and drink plenty of water.

Easy-to-wear attire: To make nursing on the road simpler, dress in cosy, nursing-friendly apparel.

NOTE If storing expressed breast milk is necessary, carry a cooler bag filled with ice packs.

Feeding Formula

Bring the necessities:

Enough formula: Determine the amount of formula your child will need for the length of your trip, plus an additional supply in case of delays.

Nipples and bottles: Bring plenty of each for every feeding. Cleaning bottles in between feedings requires the use of a bottle brush and soap.

Bring a thermos filled with hot water if you're using

powdered formula so you can quickly mix it on the move.

Insulated bottle carrier: To maintain the proper temperature for prepared bottles as required.

Get Ready in Advance: For simplicity, put pre measured formula packages or pre measured portions of formula into separate containers.

Availability: Whether in a separate travel pack or a nappy bag, make sure formula and feeding supplies are always close at hand while travelling.

Stay Clean: To avoid contamination, carefully wash your hands before handling bottles or making formula.

Be Ready for Security Inspections: Be mindful of TSA policies if you're travelling by air about bringing infant food and formula through security checks. If it becomes essential, notify security personnel and pack these goods in a different bag.

Maintain Your Schedule: To keep your baby happy and comfortable when travelling, make every effort to stick to their feeding schedule.

Whether you're formula feeding or nursing on the move, you can guarantee a more seamless travel experience by organising ahead of time and taking your baby's requirements into account.

CONCLUSION: Parenting Lifestyle Tips

Stay Organised with a Baby Tracker App

A baby tracker app can be a life-changing tool for new parents. It offers features such as feeding, diaper changes, sleep tracking, growth tracking and mood tracking. The app can help establish a routine for feeding, diaper changes and sleep, ensuring consistency in the early months of parenting.

Sharing access to the app with partners or caregivers ensures everyone is on the same page and can contribute to tracking the baby's activities.

The app also allows users to set reminders for feeding, diaper changes or nap times, which can be helpful during sleep-deprived early days. It also tracks developmental milestones and growth, providing a reference for paediatrician appointments and monitoring progress.

Health trends can be monitored by noting unusual patterns in feeding, sleeping or behaviour, which can be valuable when discussing concerns with a paediatrician. Some apps allow users to share data directly with their paediatrician or healthcare provider, facilitating communication and keeping everyone involved in the baby's care informed.

Regular data backups, either through cloud syncing or manual backups are essential to prevent data loss in case of device or technical issues. Additional features like breastfeeding timers, growth percentiles and community forums can enhance the parenting experience.

Flexibility is important when tracking a baby's activities, as every baby is different and needs to be adjusted based on their needs and cues. By staying organised with a baby tracker app, new parents can streamline their parenting responsibilities and ensure their baby is happy, healthy and well-cared for.

Take Care of Yourself Too and Involve Your Partner in Baby Care.

It may be quite taxing to care for a newborn or baby, both physically and mentally. In the bustle of feedings, changing diapers, and restless nights, it's easy for parents to overlook their own health. To maintain a positive and harmonious family dynamic, parents must prioritise self-care and engage their spouses in infant care.

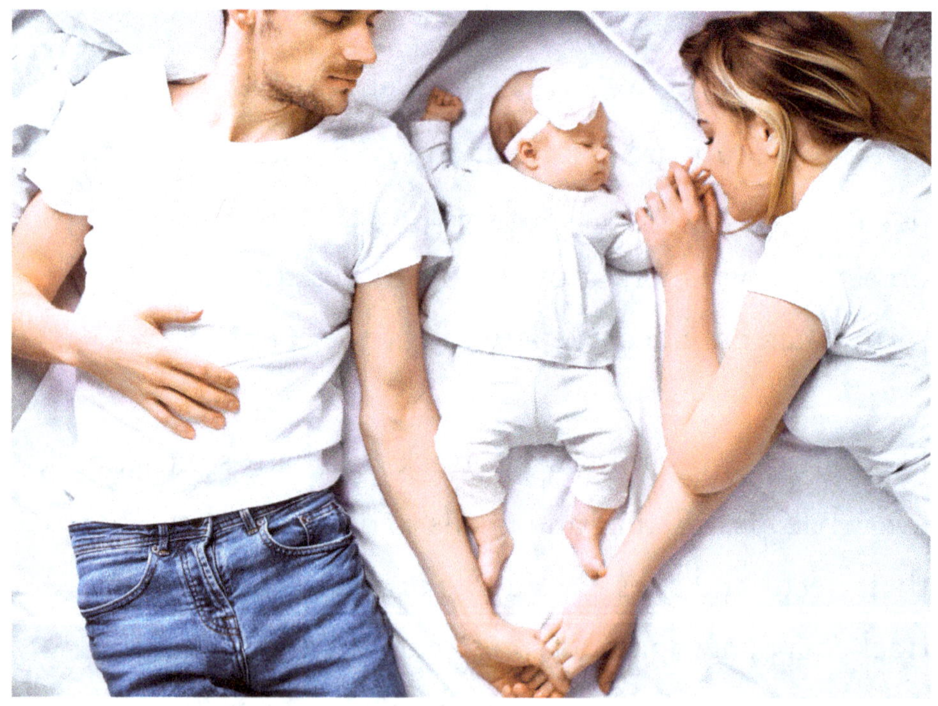

Here are some pointers for recently weds:

Rest while the baby naps: New parents often experience sleep loss, but it's important to give rest first priority whenever it can be achieved. When the baby is napping throughout the day, try to take a nap or ask relatives or friends to monitor the baby while you get your rest.

Consume wholesome meals: Eating a balanced diet is crucial for your physical and emotional wellbeing, particularly in the postpartum phase. Eat well-balanced meals and drink plenty of water throughout the day.

Accept aid: Never be reluctant to accept help from friends, family or hired help. Letting others assist with food preparation, washing or even just babysitting while you take a breather may help reduce some of the stress associated with raising a newborn.

Talk to your spouse: As a new parent, it's important to be transparent with your partner about your wants, worries and obligations. Discuss how to help each other during this trying period as you divide the burden of newborn care.

Take frequent pauses to unwind and rejuvenate, both for yourself and your companion. Taking time for yourself, whether it be by reading a book, taking a stroll or engaging in a pastime, is essential for preserving your mental health.

Remain social: Being a parent may be lonely, particularly for newly weds who may have to spend a lot of time at home taking care of their infant. Strive to maintain relationships with loved ones, friends and support networks in order to fight feelings of isolation and loneliness.

Seek expert assistance if necessary: Don't be afraid to ask a doctor or therapist for assistance if you're feeling stressed, sad, or overwhelmed. It is essential to give priority to your mental health since anxiety and postpartum depression are prevalent but curable problems.

Assign duties: Assist your spouse with all areas of caring for your child, such as feedings, changing diapers and setting up bedtimes. In addition to easing the workload for both parents, sharing responsibility promotes cooperation and a feeling of team spirit.

Spend time hugging, putting skin to skin, chatting or singing to your kid to strengthen your relationship with them. These times not only improve the relationship between parents and children, but they also provide beneficial chances for unwinding and relieving stress.

Looking after yourself is essential to becoming the best parent you can be for your child—it is not selfishness. You may provide a caring and encouraging atmosphere for your expanding family by putting self-care first and enlisting your partner's help with babysitting.

Find Support from Other Parents and Remember - This Too Shall Pass

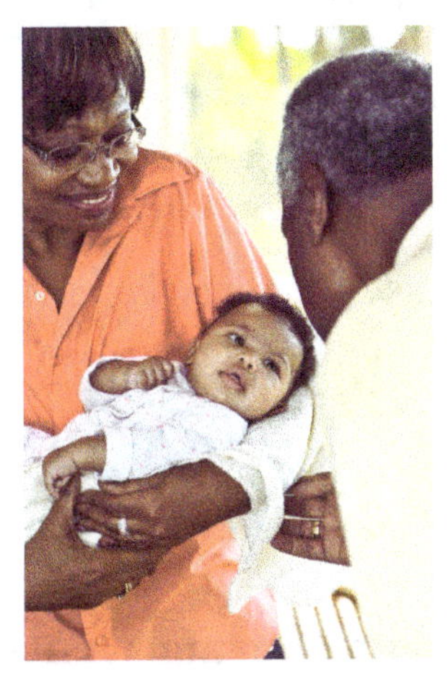

New parents can find valuable support from other parents through various methods. These include joining local parenting groups, attending parenting classes, participating in online forums and support groups, attending local parenting events, joining playgroups, using parenting apps, taking parenting classes and reaching out to friends and family members.

Parenting groups can be found on websites like **Meetup.com** or social media platforms, offering meetups, playdates and forums for discussion and support.

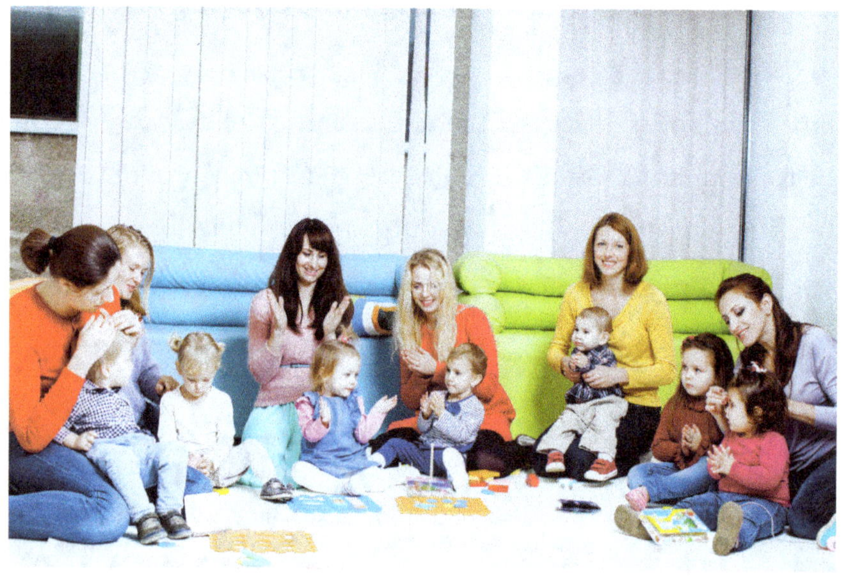

Classes can provide valuable skills and information from professionals, while online forums and support groups offer platforms for parents to ask questions and share stories.

Local parenting events, such as libraries, community centres and organisations, offer opportunities for parents to connect and support each other.

Playgroups provide an opportunity for parents and their children to socialise, while parenting apps offer features like forums, messaging and event listings to facilitate communication and support among parents.

Taking parenting classes or workshops can introduce parents to other parents seeking knowledge and support, particularly in topics like breastfeeding, infant CPR or baby care.

Note that every parent goes through challenges and struggles, but it's important to keep a positive outlook and remember that **"this too shall pass"** to navigate parenthood with grace and resilience.

Have a fantastic journey as a parent. Check out ["PREGNANT AND GOING STRONG: Exercise And Activities Guide For All 3 Trimesters,"](#) our publication.

www.ingramcontent.com/pod-product-compliance
Lightning Source LLC
Chambersburg PA
CBHW051836250726
48659CB00005B/1861